RELIEVE
YOUR ACHING HEAD

ANNE HUNT
Edited by Eric Mein, M.D.

A Note to the Reader

The information in this book is not presented as prescription for the treatment of disease. Application of the medical information found in the Edgar Cayce readings and interpreted herein should be undertaken only under the supervision of a physician.

Other Books in This Series

HEALTHY FOR LIFE: Basics for Healthy Living

MAKING JOINT DECISIONS: Preventing and Relieving Arthritis Pain

SAVING YOUR SKIN: Secrets of Healthy Skin and Hair

WEIGHT NO MORE: A Weight-Loss Program That Can Work

WINNING THE COLD WAR: Preventing and Curing the Common Cold and Flu

First Printing: May, 1992
Printed in the U.S.A.

Table of Contents

Know that there is within each individual all healing that may be accomplished for the body.　　　　　　Based on reading 4021-1

EDGAR CAYCE
PIONEER IN HOLISTIC HEALTH CARE

PREFACE

It's no secret that our society is in the midst of a health care crisis. The problem is partly economic, as we struggle to find ways to pay for the high level of care made possible by medical technology. It's also a research crisis, as scientists look for cures to diseases such as AIDS. Those are the sorts of problems that make the headlines. Those are the challenges that are clearly evident.

But our health care crisis has more subtle features, too—aspects that are easy to miss but just as important. For example, how much guarantee can doctors give us for our health? How much responsibility are we willing to accept for ourselves? Are there some ailments for which self-care is not only more economical but also more likely to produce the results we want?

Another elusive feature of our society's health care crisis is in our attitude toward health and healing itself. Recent decades have seen an explosion of alternative health services, many of them claiming to follow a more natural or a more holistic approach.

The success of some of these new methods makes us wonder about the validity of the familiar medical model. Is the body really more or less a machine that gets fixed like a balky appliance or a malfunctioning vehicle? Or is the human being a rich, complex mixture of body, mind, and spirit where problems at one level must be addressed at all three?

Working in the first four-and-a-half decades of the twentieth century, Edgar Cayce was a tremendous resource that we can now draw upon to meet the modern crisis in health care. His approach and methods for health maintenance and healing feature self-care that is often, yet not always, in conjunction with a physician's guidance. He was truly a pioneer of the contemporary holistic health movement and ahead of his time in pointing out the attitudinal, emotional, and spiritual components of disease.

Although best known as a "psychic" (or "the sleeping prophet," referring to his occasional predictions about world conditions), Cayce might be better labeled as a "clairvoyant diagnostician" or an "intuitive physician." The point with these descriptive terms is to emphasize first that Cayce's work was principally diagnostic and prescriptive. He was not a healer nor did he have office hours to see patients the way a doctor would. The cases that he took, the people who came to him for help were almost invariably those who had unsuccessfully tried the traditional medical approaches of their day and came to Cayce as a last resort, asking "What's really wrong with me? What treatments—no matter how unusual—will bring relief and healing?"

But as the descriptive labels for Cayce also emphasize, his method of meeting those requests was intuitive. He had no formal medical school training. Yet he was apparently able to alter his consciousness in such a way that he could see clairvoyantly the real origins of afflictions (physical, mental, and spiritual). What's more, he could then prescribe natural and holistic treatment procedures—sometimes requiring the involvement of a physician or other health-care professional, but often needing only a self-care regimen.

The material came through as lengthy discourses (called "readings"), which were stenographically recorded and then transcribed. Most of the information was given for specific individuals and their afflictions, but on occasion there were readings given on particular health topics which contained universally applicable information.

This book is one of a series of volumes in which common ailments and health difficulties are directed. Each topic addresses information given by Cayce which is principally focused upon self-care. The author, Anne Hunt, has carefully researched those readings on the respective health concern, focusing on the treatment procedures that were suggested to many different people as well as those recommendations that were clearly indicated for general use. Her research compilation and writing go a long way toward making these helpful methods accessible to us all. You'll find all the books in the series highly readable and very practical.

Anne's collaborator is Dr. Eric Mein, who served

as medical editor. Sometimes Cayce's language requires the insight of a trained physician to translate concepts into modern terminology. Often there are new findings in medical research that shed light on Cayce's ideas. Eric has skillfully added that dimension to the creation of this book.

This volume deals with the most common of health ailments: headaches. They are so widespread a difficulty—so universal a malady—that the term has become almost synonymous with the word "problem." For example, we might catch ourselves saying, "I've got all kinds of headaches at the office" or "That old car of mine has really become a headache." This curious facet of our language patterns reveals just how significant a role actual, physical headaches play in daily living. Ranging from minor annoyances to debilitating migraines, headaches are at least occasionally a fact of life for most people.

Perhaps no other illness tempts us more to rely exclusively on short-term, temporary treatment. It's so easy simply to take a couple of aspirin and expect four hours of relief. But masking the pain doesn't deal with the causes that may be deeper and in need of attention. As with virtually every human ailment, Cayce's approach is holistic: engaging not only the entire body as an integrated system, but also focusing on the mental and spiritual components that may contribute. After reading this book, you may still have days when pills are a remedy you turn to when a headache strikes. But you'll also be able to follow a more comprehensive approach that can lead to relief and lasting health. The Cayce readings don't claim to have *the* answer to this health dilemma, but they do offer a highly practical, self-care approach to overall prevention as well as treatment.

Mark Thurston, Ph.D.
Association for Research and Enlightenment, Inc.

INTRODUCTION

We can all relate to the discomfort of headaches, as they are one of the most common causes of pain that afflicts us. Headaches cause much suffering, an enormous loss of work-days; they adversely affect the sufferer's quality of life. For the three percent who have to deal with daily headaches or the one out of ten who has a significant headache at least weekly, any help in understanding their origins and facilitating their disappearance would be most welcome.

This book contains a unique and holistic approach to the problem of headaches. The suggestions found within these pages are based on readings given by Edgar Cayce, one of the foremost psychics of the twentieth century. The majority of his readings dealt with the physical concerns of individuals who sought his advice.

The overall approach of the Cayce source was that our bodies are intricate living "ecosystems," composed of more than seventy trillion cells, striving together to achieve harmony and health. The Cayce readings cited the ability of our cells and bodies to renew or regenerate themselves as the most fundamental of universal laws applying to our physical bodies. Health can only emerge as we provide our cells with an optimal environment by meeting their nutritional needs, clearing their waste products and other toxins, giving them coordinated messages from our nervous system, and the incentive to renew themselves from our endocrine glands. Problems arise when the component parts cannot work in harmony, leading to imbalance and dis-ease.

The Cayce approach to headaches emerges from this perspective. A person prone to frequent headaches has one or more body systems in distress, leaning them in that direction. Most commonly, this involves the elimination system, particularly the colon. The net effect of these changes creates a condition within the nervous system in which there is a lowered threshold to any stimuli. Once this has been created, any physical or mental aggravation causes a discharge of the autonomic nervous system, overstimulating the sensory system and producing the headache.

Recent research is supportive of this viewpoint. Attempts to explain migraines as being caused by a single mechanism have all failed. In addition, individuals with chronic headaches show a generalized increase in pain sensitivity to pressure and thermal pain everywhere— not just in their cranial region. Studies are also showing that head pain cannot be separated neatly into vascular and muscular origins, but that all headaches contain aspects of both along the spectrum of possibilities.

Finally, there is now good evidence that the autonomic nervous system plays an important role in the process, and that other potentiators exert their effects through its activity.

Treatment then should be aimed at restoring balance and relaxing the system. Like a garden, our bodies will respond to proper cultivation and nutrients. Such gentle coaxing enables our ecosystem to produce its best fruit, allowing not only for decreased pain, but for the enhancement of our entire experience— spiritually, mentally, and physically. The therapies suggested by the Cayce readings include osteopathic adjustments, colonics, antacids, attention to diet, and working on attitudes and emotions. As you read about this approach, much of it will make common sense, but some of the unique therapies will surprise you. At this time, more work is needed to explore the entire approach and to validate it scientifically.

As you explore these concepts, remember that the bottom line is function—the ability to move and be creative in the three dimensions in which we live. The Cayce readings invite us not only to consider their perspective, but also to put it to the test. Rather than automatically accepting their approach, we are to apply and continue to use those concepts we find helpful. To that end, enjoy this book and work with its suggestions as you continue your journey to health.

Eric Mein, M.D.
Meridian Institute

Chapter 1

HEAD FIRST?

A HAZARD OF BEING HUMAN

As we go through life, we come to accept that there are some minor and other major ailments that will crop up here and there along the way. Stomach aches and common colds are universally accepted as two of the potential pitfalls of being human. Running right beside these common ailments—if not ahead of them—are headaches: those nagging aches which range from minor irritations to debilitating pains. They often demand as much courage, backbone, and positive thinking as we can muster.

HOW HEADACHES HAPPEN

Headaches are a unique form of illness in that the symptoms are frequently simple and straightforward. The pain may be sharp, or it may be dull. It may

1

seem to haunt your whole head, or it may seem focused in one area. Sometimes your neck stiffens and adds to your distress. Be that as it may, it is still pain—in the head—which sends you seeking relief.

And with simple headaches relief is often easily found. Since headaches can lack the complexity of aches and pains of a cold or flu, you usually don't have to deal all at once with a multitude of symptoms. There's no sore throat complicated by fever. You're not fighting congestion while suffering from fatigue. Thus, in the case of minor and infrequent headaches, there is a temptation to simply head to the medicine chest for an aspirin and then off to bed for relief. Even severe headaches, if relatively irregular, are often accepted with stoicism, a pain reliever, and rest.

If we spend any time at all pondering the origins of our aching head and neck, we often conclude that stress, lack of sleep, or poor eating habits are the culprits. Our thoughts tend to stop with these casual reflections—and move on to the most immediate avenue for relief. Again, a pain reliever and rest.

But your interest in this book indicates a desire to understand your head and neck ache syndromes more fully. What exactly are the pains in your head? What causes them? Can they be prevented? And if prevention fails, can they be relieved?

You'll find the answers to these questions in the following chapters. Though you'll discover that headaches may be caused by a number of complex imbalances within your body systems, you'll be relieved to find that preventative measures are surprisingly simple. And, in many instances, these same preventative therapies and principles can also be mobilized for relief.

The basic premise of this book is that headaches, like all forms of illness, can best be prevented and cured through a holistic approach to health and healing; that means, by treating your *self* as an integration of body, mind, and soul. Holism discounts treating a pain with a pill as the best option for health. It challenges you to view yourself as a spiritual being, programmed for health, destined for wholeness. It empowers you to awaken the healer within to strengthen body, mind, and soul.

One of the most recognized and respected sources for holistic advice about physical ailments is Edgar Cayce. Among the wealth of materials he imparted through his clairvoyant diagnoses was information on headaches, information which was and is uniquely insightful and refreshingly practical. You'll find that information in this book.

But first, before we move on to prevention and cure of headaches, let's examine the phenomenon itself.

A HISTORY OF HEADACHES

In all likelihood, headaches have plagued humankind since the beginning of time. For thousands of years physicians and practitioners have studied headaches, tried to understand their origins, and attempted to find relief for sufferers. Traditionally, two major categories of headaches have been isolated, distinguished primarily by the hypothesized physiological, immediate causes of the pain. In some cases, this was felt to involve muscular tension and stress; in others, swelling and abnormally functioning blood vessels were felt to be the culprits. Research now indicates that there is a significant amount of overlap between these two causes of headaches and that an altered balance of the nervous system is behind both. However, it still can be useful to discuss them individually.

TENSION HEADACHES

The most common form of headache is associated with muscular tension in the neck, jaw, face, eyes, ears, and mouth. There are well over thirty individual muscles regulating head and neck movement, facial expressions, talking, chewing, looking, even laughing. These muscles can become tense for dozens of reasons. Some are obvious—squinting in bright light, tightening your jaw under duress, leaning over your desk all day. Other causes for muscular tension are less obvious. Spinal misalignment can cause muscular strain in the head and neck. Toxins within your system can have a tensing effect upon your muscles. And so can lack of sleep, irregular exercise, even poor nutrition!

The result is a dull, aching head.

VASCULAR HEADACHES

The more severe and often more serious type of headaches are thought to involve abnormal vascular tone. For a variety of physiological reasons, blood vessels in the head first constrict and then quickly dilate, putting pressure on nearby nerves.

Migraine headaches fall into this category and can seem relentless in terms of degree of pain and long-term reoccurrence. Migraines most often seem to affect half the head and cause sharp, throbbing pain. Medical science offers several theories as to the causes of migraines, including hypoglycemia, poor diet, stress. In many cases, however, the sufferer never really pinpoints the cause and thus never experiences a cure. The symptoms are usually treated with pain relievers. In many cases, a vicious cycle of pain and pills continues throughout life.

There are other forms of vascular headaches as well. The swelling of blood vessels due to high blood pressure is one. Another is withdrawal from stimulants such as caffeine. Sinus infections, overexertion, and certain medications and food additives can all cause headaches. And, we can't overlook the infamous hangover headache. Finally, headaches caused by toxic substances in the blood can cause abnormalities in the functioning of the arterial circulation.

The result in all cases is sharp and often throbbing pain.

BE SMART

Though most headaches are self-limiting and seem to fall neatly into the tension or vascular categories, it is important to realize that head pain is not always caused by isolated muscular and/or vascular stress. If at any time you experience abnormal or unusual head and neck pain, especially if it is associated with fever or stiff neck, or is pain that is greatest at night or on first arising, see your physician at once. Because, though headaches may seem to be simply a hazard of being human, sometimes they are signals of other serious problems. It is smart to be sure of the origins of any head pain.

A UNIQUE PERSPECTIVE

The Cayce readings recognize the same immediate physiological causes of head and neck aches as medical science. Muscles can become tender and tense, blood vessels can become swollen, and pain can result. But the readings offer tremendous insight into the *underlying* causes for these conditions. The bottom line of this insight is simple.

Over a period of time, a number of factors combine to create a lowered stimulation threshold within the nervous system. Eventually, *anything that can react adversely on the nervous, circulatory, or digestive system may ultimately cause a headache.*

Fortunately for the headache sufferer, these systems can be brought under your control. Though there is no quick panacea to gain such command when things have gone awry, there are simple principles of health that, when applied consistently, can help bring your body's vital systems into balance. And, as mentioned earlier, these same basic health principles pack powerful preventative medicine as well.

But before we begin to discuss prevention and cure, let's take a look at what specific causes Cayce revealed for both tension and migraine headaches. These insights will help you understand your condition better, and thus position you to embark upon the road to recovery with greater speed and more chance for success.

Chapter 2

CLOSE-UP ON
TENSION HEADACHES

CAYCE ON TENSION HEADACHES

Tension headaches are perhaps more common than the common cold. They can result from stresses as different as an angry boss and excessive mental stress to fatigue, poor diet, and eyestrain. Though tension headaches have been traditionally characterized by medical science as generally muscular in nature, Cayce was ahead of his time viewing them as a combination of muscular and vascular disorders. He went on to say that they originated from imbalances within the nervous, circulatory, or digestive systems of the body.

When one is suffering from a headache and trying to cure it, whether it is due to muscular contractions or abnormalities within the vascular system becomes a mute point. What is important is the root cause of the pain . . . where it originates and how it can be corrected.

You're about to read Cayce's specific insights into tension headaches. First, you'll learn probable causes; then, you'll come to understand possible cures. And, hopefully needed only as an interim measure, you'll learn some natural pain relief techniques to help you get through the headache attack.

PROBABLE CAUSES

In the most general terms, Cayce indicated that the root cause of most headaches was not in the head but elsewhere in the body. As discussed earlier, anything that can have an adverse effect upon the nervous, circulatory, or digestive system can result in reflex muscular and vascular stress, producing a headache. Since these three systems depend so upon one another, if one gets upset, the others soon follow suit. Havoc wreaked on the body can shoot straight to the head.

General Debilitation When your body is run down, you're at risk of developing general fatigue and subsequent head pain. Simply put, your body doesn't have the energy and resources it needs to maintain proper health. Your digestion can become disturbed, your circulation sluggish. Probably you know that "run down" feeling all too well. The result is an overtoxic system and poor circulation to the head. Headaches often result.

Excessive Mental and Emotional Strain Cayce offered interesting insights into how mental and emotional stress could result in headaches. In short, he indicated that such stress adversely affects the nervous, circulatory, and digestive systems. Think for a moment the last time you had an argument and tried to eat afterward. The result may well have been lack of appetite or indigestion. Your anger or feelings of being upset may well have sent your blood pressure soaring. You may have even felt "nervous" as a result of the encounter. In other words, you've directly experienced how stress can affect your digestion, circulation, and nerves! And all of these feelings can translate to your head!

Nervous System Disorders Interestingly, Cayce indicated that an overtaxation or incoordination of the nervous system could affect nerve impulses to certain parts of the body, including the head. According to Cayce's description of this unfortunate chain of events, this condition could alter the balance of nerve impulses, causing abnormal muscular contractions, which could lead to headaches, fatigue, and even vertigo.

To understand this concept better, think of the electrical system in your car. These electrical impulses operate your headlights, windshield wipers, radio, and all other electrical devices. If the electrical system is overtaxed or "injured," it blows a fuse! And then, whatever device that fuse supported ceases to function properly—or altogether! That's the way your spinal system works as well. If it is overtaxed in some way, the nerve impulses it normally transmits, whether to your colon or your circulatory system, can be affected, overstimulating some areas while "blowing a fuse" in others.

Digestive Disorders A build-up of mucus and toxins in the digestive tract was often targeted as a condition which could ultimately result in headaches. Why? A build-up of toxins would result in a release of these wastes *into* the system (rather than *out* of it!), causing general stress on all systems within the body. The readings in particular discuss both the stomach and colon as playing a role in this process. In addition, a disorder of the digestive tract could result in poor assimilation of nutrients, causing fatigue and low energy. As we've discussed before, headaches could be the result of such disorder.

Circulatory Disorders Your circulatory system is actually made up of two distinct systems—the arterial and lymph systems. The arterial system delivers nutrients to every cell of your body, while the lymph system picks up the waste by-products of each cell's daily functioning. Your circulatory system relies heavily upon the health of other bodily systems for its own well-being.

In the case of headaches, Cayce saw circulatory problems as arising from an overacid condition in the digestive tract, compounded by poor assimilation of nutrients. The bloodstream, then, becomes toxic and nutrient poor. Thus, it cannot properly nourish muscular tissue nor can the lymph deal effectively with the excess toxic wastes. The result, as with all other imbalances described previously, could well be a headache and fatigue.

Eyestrain   Although eyestrain was not frequently mentioned by Cayce as a major cause of headaches, it was periodically the culprit. In some cases, the eyestrain was caused by difficulties in focusing at close range and at a distance. The muscular stresses this caused could put pressure on the optic nerve, resulting in often sharp and uncomfortable headaches.

SUGGESTED THERAPIES

Where to Begin

If you suffer from frequent headaches, the following suggestions will be of help. You'll want to begin with the basics, correcting your diet and improving your eliminations while integrating other health-promoting therapies and activities into your life style. Here's what you need to know to get started:

Review Your Diet   Diet is such an integral part of health that it is always wise to assess and review your eating habits when haunted by headache pain (or any other pain for that matter). In short, you want to correct any overacidity in your digestive tract, start to assimilate nutrients better, and build your blood so that it is rich and nourishing to the rest of your body. Chapter 5 tells you everything you need to know to correct and improve your diet.

Consider an Antacid   An antacid may seem to be an unusual suggestion for headache sufferers, but the readings often made this suggestion. If you discover that your system is overacid (see *Appendix D*) or you have problems with indigestion or gas after meals, take a mild antacid to correct the problem.

The most frequent antacid suggested by Cayce was Al-Caroid, an antacid which is no longer on the market. However, a substitute mentioned in the readings was bisodol, which can now be found in tablet form. Cayce suggested its use after the heaviest meal of the day. This rather simple compound packs quite a punch in terms of benefits to your digestive system. First and foremost, it helps combat overacidity, stimulates assimilation, and improves eliminations. It's a good remedy to have on your shelf in case you're ever in need.

Get a Spinal Adjustment Spinal adjustments were often recommended as a part of headache therapy. The reason is simple. They directly help restore health and balance to your nervous system. In the case of headaches, osteopaths were suggested as the preferable professional to administer these adjustments. An osteopath can concentrate on restoring an even, normal flow of nerve impulses throughout your spinal column. As a result, your nervous system better directs your body's activities—from digestion to circulation. An added bonus, a relaxed healthy spine can result in relaxed and healthy muscles—especially in the back, neck, and head area.

How can you best begin this therapy? Simply find an osteopath who practices manual medicine and with whom you feel comfortable; discuss your needs. Cayce suggested a series of treatments like this. Get one to two adjustments a week for three weeks. Leave off a week. Then repeat this series. Your osteopath will help you set up a series of sessions which address your individual problems. You may well be surprised at how helpful this therapy can be.

Cope More Effectively with Mental and Emotional Stress As discussed earlier, mental and emotional stress can result in nervous incoordination, poor digestion, even sluggish circulation. Unfortunately, stress is a part of everyday life, whether it be in the form of traffic jams or personal finances! How, then, can it be removed?

The idea is not to try to remove stress altogether because trying to do so in today's world is impossible! The best approach to stress is to learn to cope in more positive ways. This is such an important part of headache therapy that Chapter 6 is devoted to "attitude adjusters," a series of stress-reducers you can incorporate into your daily life. Basically, they are aimed at helping you work with your subconscious mind to find new sources of peace and comfort in an often hectic world. Of all the chapters in this book, it is the most important one. Be sure to read it—and practice it as well.

Clean Your Colon As you know, Cayce focused on problems in the intestinal tract as possible causes of headaches. Whether you have a mucous or toxic build-up (or both!), your head may well be the ultimate victim. Why? Because your colon is vital in the elimination process. If disturbed, fatigue and nervous disorders can result.

Obviously, an improved diet which includes high-fiber content will help cleanse your colon. But, sometimes diet alone isn't enough. You'll want to consider a good "colon cleansing," either via a series of colonics administered by a professional therapist or by giving yourself a series of enemas at home. In the case of headaches, Cayce suggested that you might begin with two colon cleansings in the first three weeks you undertake your therapy. Afterward, simply take them often enough to keep your colon free of mucus and toxins, perhaps monthly.

Refer to *Appendix D* to learn how to administer an enema.

Get a Massage A regular massage can be a vital part of building better circulation and improving your eliminations. As with any medical professional, try to find a massage therapist whom you feel comfortable with and pursue a regular routine. Discuss your headache problems when you begin your visits, and suggest that your therapist concentrate on your spinal and cranial area.

Or, if you are unable to visit a massage therapist, get in the habit of a "self-massage" as described in *Appendix D*. Whichever you choose, you'll want to select carefully the type of oil with which you're massaged. In the case of headaches as well as many other common ailments, Cayce recommended an equal mixture of olive and peanut oil as a good massage oil.

Use an Electrical Vibrator An electrical vibrator was suggested in hundreds of Cayce's readings for a variety of ailments. Headaches were among them. Electrical vibrators are available through distributors of health supplies as well as through many department stores. A general approach for applying the vibrator is to use it along the entire cerebrospinal system just before retiring. The result is a more relaxed nervous system. Though the readings stress that this therapy does not correct the causes behind the disrupted nervous system, it does offer temporary correction and relief.

When shopping for your vibrator, find one with a cup or suction attachment. You can use this device to massage the area just above the diaphragm. This will help stimulate digestion and assimilation, which can in turn help prevent and relieve headache pain.

Rest Your Eyes   If you feel that eyestrain is involved in your headaches, be sure to rest your eyes periodically, perhaps covering them with a cool cloth. You may find this to be a nice routine when you get ready for bed, especially after a hectic day. And, be sure to practice the "head and neck" exercise described in Chapter 6—both mornings and evenings. Not only will this exercise help correct the effects of eyestrain, it is also good for minor ear problems, including tinnitus (ringing in the ears). This exercise was suggested for eye *and* ear care in hundreds of Cayce's readings. Why not benefit from this advice yourself?

NATURAL PAIN RELIEVERS

Unfortunately, whatever preventative measures you employ, you may still fall prey to headache pain. It is hoped that these will be with decreasing frequency and intensity than before. When in the throes of a headache, there are a few common-sense steps

16

to take for relief. Though they may sound as if they're right out of your grandmother's medicine chest, they still can have the much-needed soothing effects you desire.

Take Time Out   Since many of the underlying causes of headaches have to do with mental and physical stress, rest is the number-one therapy for relief. When headache pain begins, it's important to get some rest as soon as possible. If the pain is minor, a few moments of time out of a hectic day may just do the trick. If your discomfort is more severe, you may want to take time out for an hour or two and find a quiet place to lie down and rest. If you do . . .

Cover Your Eyes with a Cold Cloth   On several occasions Cayce recommended covering your eyes with a cool cloth as a way to disperse some of those headache pains. And don't think a cool cloth over your eyes is only possible in the privacy of your home. If a headache comes on while you're at work, take a short break with a damp cloth and lay your head back in a comfortable position. Those few moments may help relieve your pain and give you a calmer perspective on the rest of your day. Relax!

Soothe Your Temples   A special remedy was suggested for one individual with headaches; it was encouraged to be used while resting with a cool cloth over the eyes. Mix together equal parts of camphor and tincture of lobelia, both of which can be found at many natural food stores. Rub this compound into the

17

temples, just before lying down to rest. Its soothing effects may surprise you.

Get a Massage As you know massage can be beneficial in the long-term treatment of headache pain. But it was often suggested as a pain relief therapy. If your headache is severe, see if you can arrange for a massage. Being rubbed the right way at the right time might just spell relief.

Take an Antacid. An antacid can also help bring short-term relief from head pain. See the previous discussion on pages 12 and 13.

Take a Bath—If You Can One person was told to take a series of three hot and cold alternating baths to help relieve headache pain. You might want to take alternating hot and cold showers for ease. Sound like an odd suggestion. Well, it may well be. However, it is an easy pain reliever to try. If it works for you, you'll be glad to have it in your repertoire of remedies.

Mental Muscle Relaxers Whatever pain relievers you select, remember to rest your mind as you treat your body. Whether it is soft music or peace and quiet which provides the best atmosphere for you, seek it out. Then free your mind of the worries and stresses of the day. Try breathing deeply and regularly, breathing in peace and calm with every breath, breathing out stress as you exhale. If worries or concerns creep in, gently guide your mind to pleasant thoughts. Getting your mind off your day's worries will relax you and allow your physical therapies to work.

Chapter 3

CLOSE-UP ON MIGRAINES

CAYCE ON MIGRAINES

Anyone who has suffered from migraine pain knows how debilitating an attack can be and how worrisome the fear of an unexpected attack. Many people have sought treatment for these recurring headaches—only to find that treatments often end up being aimed at the symptoms, rather than at the elusive underlying causes. Cayce's perspective on migraines was as unique as his overall approach to headache pain. Like his overall approach, Cayce saw migraines as a symptom of other internal imbalances.

You're about to read about Cayce's specific insights into migraine headaches. First, you'll learn probable causes; then, you'll come to understand possible cures. And, hopefully needed only as an interim measure, you'll be referred again to some natural pain relief techniques.

CAUSES

Cayce revealed a multitude of internal imbalances which could lead to a migraine condition. They are listed below. It is important to reiterate that Cayce viewed all body systems as interdependent upon one another. Thus, when one of the following problems developed, it would be highly likely that one or more of the others would soon follow.

Poor Eliminations   Our elimination systems consist of our skin, colon, kidneys and liver, and lungs. In women, menstrual periods also serve a role in the elimination process. All are responsible for the disposal of spent material from our bodies—whether they be internally generated as our bodies burn energy or externally imported as we eat, breathe, and expose our skin to external substances. However, if not properly functioning, our elimination systems can trap and absorb toxins, rather than sending them on their way! Overtoxicity can have a tremendous impact upon both the circulatory and nervous systems. The risk is simple. Poor eliminations can result in head pain.

Congestion in the Colon   Of the possible problems with eliminations, Cayce most commonly pinpointed colon congestion as a cause of migraines. In other words, it was the unique condition which, when developed, triggered the migraine. In this chain of events, Cayce felt that mucous congestion and adhesions in the colon created pressures on the autonomic nervous system and certain portions of the spine.

These, in turn, reflexively affected the trigeminal or 5th cranial nerve and cranial circulation, resulting in vascular headaches.

But, what causes the colon congestion? Here we see the interdependence of bodily systems once again. Poor diet, glandular imbalance, poor assimilation, and nervous stress can all play a role in producing congestion of your digestive system.

Incoordination of the Nervous Systems Our cerebrospinal system consists of our brain and our spinal cord. It functions as a "higher mind" to our autonomic nervous system which usually operates involuntarily—directing our organs' activities and maintaining internal harmony within our body. Together, these nervous systems are responsible for directing our body's many and varied activities, both conscious and unconscious. Thus, it is not surprising that poor team play between these two systems can wreak havoc on our health.

Among the many tasks our autonomic nervous systems perform is the regulation of blood vessels and blood flow. It also plays a role in tissue inflammation. It is not surprising, then, that when it is out of kilter, vascular headaches (of which migraines reign as king!) can result.

Poor Assimilation When your body loses or lessens its ability to absorb nutrients, it becomes run-down and overtaxed. It simply does not have the resources it needed to be healthy and whole. A direct effect of poor assimilation is a depletion of the body energies needed to maintain the nervous and circulatory systems

21

at their prime. Cayce cited stomach problems as producing a reflex through the vagus nerve that can lead to headaches. He also said that food allergies can play a role in some individuals, especially adolescents.

Poor Circulation   Poor circulation seldom happens in and of itself—as is obvious from the above discussions. Think of the vast network of vessels leading to and nourishing your head and neck areas. To get a clear picture of this intricate network of arteries and veins, refer to an anatomy book in your local library. Disturbances in blood flow and pressure can have obvious results.

As your circulation is disturbed, erratic modulation of blood flow can result in the sharp and throbbing pain characterized by migraines.

General Debilitation   General debilitation can be the result of any of the above conditions—or it can cause them. Your body needs an adequate supply of energy as well as adequate reserves to call upon in times of stress. All of the general health hints given throughout this book will help you maintain an even and steady energy level which will result in health and healing.

SUMMING UP

Again, the above list of possible causes of migraine headaches emphasizes that our bodies are a complex network of interdependent systems. If one is out of kilter, the others are likely to follow soon. With the system out of balance, any physical or emotional stressor can set off the chain of events leading to a headache. As discussed throughout this book, the curing of any pain or disease must take this complexity into consideration.

So where do migraine sufferers begin? What is a reasonable, health-promoting regimen of therapy to follow for relief?

SUGGESTED THERAPIES

Below are some suggestions for a series of healthful therapies to help bring balance to your body's vital systems. These suggestions are geared toward the correction of the underlying causes which may be the culprits in your migraine pain. When Cayce made the following types of suggestions, he stressed the importance of consistency and persistency in applying them. Your chances for success improve dramatically if this advice is followed.

He also made another important observation. As with many new, health-promoting activities, they sometimes make you feel worse before you feel better. Think of the last time you started a new exercise program. You probably knew the program was good for you, but on that second or third day, your body may have felt more tired and sore than before you began. Or, if you've ever dramatically changed your diet or stopped drinking coffee, you may have felt some pain before the rewarding feeling of gain. Just remember that the therapies below may well have those same effects. But don't give up! Persistency and consistency will bring a renewed sense of health to your ailing body.

Without further ado, here are therapeutic suggestions

23

specific to migraine sufferers.

Get Spinal Adjustments Consult with an osteopath who practices manual medicine regarding a series of spinal manipulations aimed at relaxing the system and restoring healthful nerve communications along your spine and throughout your body. One routine Cayce suggested was to get one or two adjustments a week for three weeks, then leave off a week, and then repeat. Maintenance adjustments may be needed every three to four months after the initial treatments. Be sure to talk with your practitioner about your headaches so that he or she is aware of your condition. That way, you'll get the best possible help to alleviate your migraine pain.

Cleanse Your Colon Cleansing the colon to remove mucus and accumulated waste is a vital step in migraine therapy. Colonics, enemas, and gentle laxatives can all play a vital role in this process. If you can find a therapist who administers colonics, you may want to choose this avenue to begin your therapy. As discussed under "Tension Headaches," a good approach to colon cleansing is to begin by cleansing the colon two times in three weeks, then often enough to maintain a toxic-free system. If you elect to administer a series of enemas, you can conveniently find instructions in *Appendix D*. And, if you would prefer to work with a gentle laxative, pure olive oil, taken in small doses—one teaspoon several times a day—is an excellent choice.

Use an Antacid Keeping your system alkaline is important in the battle against migranes. You can test your acid-alkaline balance using the instructions in *Appendix D*. If you have the need to take steps to alkalize, follow the suggestions for taking bisodol found in Chapter 2. The diet suggestions in Chapter 5 will also help you bring about a healthy acid-alkaline balance through proper food.

Apply Castor Oil Packs   Although you'll find general instructions for the use of castor oil packs to stimulate the eliminations systems in Chapter 4 and *Appendix D*, Cayce also gave specific advice for these packs in the case of migraine headaches. You should apply the packs once or twice a week over the right side of the abdomen. Keep them on for an hour to an hour-and-a-half at a time. On the following day, take two teaspoons of olive oil internally. Follow this as a weekly routine, monitoring how you feel it contributing to your progress. A series of three castor oil packs before a colonic can help increase its effectiveness as well.

Improve Your Diet   Basically, every diet can be improved, especially in today's fast-paced world! Follow the general guidelines for diet in Chapter 5. In addition, here are some important hints: Choose foods which build blood and nurture nerves. Go heavy on green leafy vegetables, fruits, and whole grains. Avoid at all costs white bread, combining starches in one meal, fried foods, sugar, red meat, and carbonated drinks. Some individuals were told specifically to avoid chocolates and other sweets. Become aware of your own reactions to certain foods and consider the possibility of a food allergy.

Administer Electrotherapy The Cayce readings viewed the body as a battery and the electricity running through it as "life." Keeping the battery "charged" was important. If it were to run down, the body would become depleted in life-giving energy. Since debilitation was one of the problems connected with migraines, electrotherapy was a part of the suggested regimen.

The type of electrotherapy most often suggested in the readings for migraines is use of the Impedance Device. The purpose of the device is to revitalize and energize the body's electrical energies which help regulate blood and nerve flow, which in turn strengthens the body and restores it to health.

You'll find directions for use of the Impedance Device in *Appendix D.*

Enjoy a Regular Massage Though not recommended in the majority of migraine readings, massage was suggested several times. One person was told to have a massage focused between the shoulders with cocoa butter following each castor oil pack (described above). Since massage is both relaxing and stimulates circulation, you may want to try it as a part of your therapy. Monitor whether you feel that it is helpful to your condition. If you have positive feelings about this therapy, continue. Remember, your body knows best.

PAIN RELIEF

Refer to the section on "Natural Pain Relievers" in Chapter 2 to find some common-sense, but helpful suggestions to help deal with migraine pain. Though it is true that these suggestions will in all likelihood fall short of stopping the migraine pain, they are better than the other alternative . . . which is medication.

A WORD ON SEDATIVES

Sedatives are often recommended by physicians to help bring relief during severe migraine attacks. Cayce recognized their practicality and necessity, yet also indicated that sedatives could have adverse effects upon the body and may well aggravate a condition rather than help alleviate it. As you begin these other therapies, try to diminish your use of the sedatives until you can comfortably discontinue them. You may also want to consult with your physician about possible alternatives that can help you taper off the sedatives at a faster rate.

Chapter 4

HEADS UP ON HEALTH

HOW HEALTH HAPPENS

Cayce's general approach to tension and migraine headaches may have raised more questions than it answered. If you are new to a holistic approach to health, you may understandably be a bit confused about how your body systems can work together with both mind and spirit to bring about health. And along with that health—a final goodbye to head and neck pain! So, without further ado, here's a primer in health and healing—the natural way!

To be healthy, you must begin to understand some basics about your miraculous body. Though you may tend to underrate your body, especially when you are experiencing pain, it is nonetheless amazing in the way it functions from day to day. Of course, it has help. This help comes in the form of your mind and your spirit.

Lasting health is the result of a partnership among body, mind, and spirit. One Cayce reading summed up this connection when it revealed that "every phase of the physical, mental and spiritual life is dependent upon the other." (2533-3)[1]

Cayce sketched a picture of the complex workings of the human being which was truly ground-breaking for his time. He identified three distinct parts which combine to make a whole person—a physical body, a mental body, and a spiritual body. In describing the relationship among these bodies, Cayce used the following powerful concept: spirit is the life, mind is the builder, and the physical is the result. In other words, we derive our life from a power greater than ourselves. We then filter this spirit through our thought patterns. And our bodies, in their turn, respond to these signals.

This is how health happens. Your spirit speaks through your mind to your body. But what exactly is your spirit? What is your mind? And how can they influence the well-being of your body?

Let's take a closer look.

SPIRIT-WISE

Within each of us is an innate wisdom that brings and renews life in our bodies. This wisdom is an

---

[1] The Edgar Cayce readings have each been assigned a two-part number for identification. The first digits indicate the specific number assigned to the topic or individual obtaining the reading. Since many received more than one reading, the second set of digits following the hyphen indicates the number in that particular series of readings.

unseen energy that gives us life. It helps us reproduce, not only through the miracle of childbirth, but also through the miracle of growth and healing. Every day our bodies regenerate and repair at the cellular level. The energy which fuels such cellular transformation also directs the complex operation of our bodies, in almost all cases without our conscious knowledge. Our hearts beat, our liver performs metabolic functions, our lungs process oxygen and release carbon dioxide. All of these activities depend on spirit in action as a renewal force working to keep our bodies functioning properly.

How is this energy, this wisdom, transmitted to the body? How does it give the right signals and directions? According to the readings, there are specific points of contact between our spiritual and physical bodies. These conductors are our endocrine glands. The readings pay special attention to seven of these glands in explaining the connection between the spiritual and the physical: the gonads, the cells of Leydig, the adrenals, the thymus, thyroid, pineal, and pituitary. These glands, along with the assistance of many other vital glands, secrete potent molecules which affect and regulate literally thousands of metabolic functions, including the regeneration of cells and tissues. It is here that our bodies interface with spirit to continue to function properly and maintain health and balance. Why, then, are our bodies so individualized and of varying degrees of health and illness? Where do we go wrong? Why do we get sick?

MIND MATTERS

Our minds are often the culprits. According to the Cayce readings, our mental bodies contain a collection of patterns which create our physical life. First, there are the genetic patterns and physiological tendencies we chose on a mental level prior to birth. What we look like, from eye color to body type, depends in great part upon our genetic coding. Second, there are the conscious and subconscious mental patterns which are constantly shaping our lives and coming to bear on our inborn tendencies. These are most easily recognized as both our attitudes and emotions and our habits. If these result in a relatively healthy, balanced life style, the physical result will, for the most part, be positive. If we exercise, our muscles will be better toned. If we get enough sleep and eat well, we will generally look more rested and healthful. Likewise, if we are negative in the way we think and act or continue unhealthy patterns of diet and exercise, there will be unpleasant side effects on our body and our health.

But what, exactly, makes our attitudes and emotions positive? What makes them negative? How do our habits form? How can they be changed?

Though we are aware of our conscious thoughts and feelings, a great deal goes on in the depths of our subconscious minds. It is here that our mental patterns play out their agendas, in large part completely hidden to us. Many of the problems we encounter in life as well as the seeming miracles that come our way originate in our subconscious mind. The texture of our mind springs from many complex sources involving our own personal histories. Childhood experiences, family influences, and events we have experienced as adults are just a few of the major foods for the subconscious. Finding positive patterns and building upon them to feed the conscious and subconscious can help us grow toward greater health.

BODY BASICS

The body you see in the mirror is a result of your mental patterns, both genetic and learned, and how these have affected your physiology. But where exactly do these patterns make their mark? On the building blocks of our bodies, our cells—of which there are over 70 trillion! Cayce indicated that each cell is a world of its own, capable of finding perfection and working in unison with other cells to reconstruct the body toward better health. To accomplish this feat of renewal and regeneration, these microcosms need to exist in an environment free of toxins, take in the proper nutrition, and receive the right signals from your mind or mental body. Given these three elements, they can slowly but surely begin to realize the perfection that gives them life and reward you with greater health and wholeness.

AHEAD OF THE GAME

If you can work with the concept of body, mind, and spirit and use it to create health, you'll find yourself ahead of the game. Don't wait until you are ill with a headache to try to retrace your steps to find out where you went wrong. Become proactive for health. Create a life style that nurtures body, mind, and spirit and stick to it. Sound difficult? Really, it's not. Here's how.

THE WISDOM WITHIN

Your body is a complex network of interdependent systems. From your digestive to your circulatory to your nervous system, your body is constantly pumping, communicating, processing, and eliminating. Good health results when these systems function as they are intended—in harmony with one another.

As you've learned, the wisdom to maintain these systems when you are in good health and to steer them to healing when you are ill lies within. This inner wisdom, however, greatly benefits from your assistance. It is your responsibility to create an environment which promotes health and healing. But where do you start? How can you possibly understand the complexities of your body's physiology so that you can care for it properly? Luckily the task is much easier than you might expect. You do not have to *tell* your body systems what, when, and why things must be done. You simply need to enhance how your systems work by taking steps that make their job easier.

The systems which are the most basic and important to your general health are those that work with assimilation, elimination, and circulation. Your nervous system serves as the conductor of this internal symphony. As you learned previously, all these systems have a particular impact upon your head. What's important for you to know is that in the same way their disharmony can cause headaches, their harmony can ward them off!

They are each affected by many of your daily activities (or inactivities!) and can, with some simple, basic care be made whole and healthy.

THE CONDUCTOR

Your nervous system acts like the conductor of a symphony orchestra in directing the activities of your body and thus must function properly if you wish to have good health. The "trunk line" of this communication system is your spinal cord. Your brain sends signals down your spinal cord, signals which are then relayed to various corners of your body via a complex communications system. If your nervous system is out of balance, the directions it sends to the members of the symphony—your organs, muscles, and other bodily tissues—can result in disorder, rather than harmony.

Nerve impulses are meant to serve many vital functions. Nerves may stimulate regeneration, growth, development, self-maintenance, and repair at the cellular level. On a larger scale, they regulate the activities of organs and glands, activate muscles, and control the body's blood supply—thus, as discussed earlier, their involvement in head pain.

Cayce targeted spinal misalignment (called "subluxations") as the cause of many of the body's ills. Likewise, Cayce revealed that it is through spinal adjustments from a trained professional that much good could be accomplished to regain equilibrium among the body's systems. Without a healthy, properly functioning nervous system, the body simply cannot maintain a high level of health, no matter how much we may nurture and promote good health through other systems, such as eliminations and circulation. To keep your spine in optimal shape and your nervous system dispatching important, life-giving signals, you should obtain regular spinal adjustments by an osteopath.

TOXIC WASTE REMOVAL

The news media is constantly full of reports about toxic waste removal and how important it is to keeping our planet healthy and whole. Our bodies can be seen as microcosms of the great macrocosm—the living earth. Just as the earth has plants to process carbon dioxide and release oxygen to keep the atmosphere clear and life supporting, we have lungs to take in oxygen and release carbon dioxide, to keep the atmosphere in our bodies clear and life supporting.

Our elimination systems serve to keep our bodies clean and free of toxins. Five major organs are involved in this important mission: the kidneys, liver, colon, lungs, and skin. Each of these organs must function properly and in harmony with the others. Thus, your daily habits and health therapies should take them individually and collectively into account. Cayce stressed the importance of eliminations when he stated: "Clear the body as you do the mind of those things that have been hindered. The things that hinder physically are the poor eliminations. Set up better eliminations in the body." (2524-5)

But what is it, exactly, that we are trying to eliminate? First, our bodies struggle to eliminate the by-products we obtain from external sources. Our food often bears dangerous additives and empty calories which must be broken down and eliminated. The air we breathe and the elements which come in contact with our skin must also be processed by our bodies with the wastes duly disposed. Many people are not aware, however, that wastes are not simply the by-products of what is taken in to the body, but also the result of internal "combustion" processes that occur on the cellular level. The day-to-day internal functioning of our cells burns energy and creates by-products, which the Cayce readings called ash. Compound this toxic build-up with the three to eight billion cells which die each day as a part of the renewal process. Thus, you begin to develop a clearer picture of the magnitude of the many and varied tasks our elimination systems face as they go about our body's housekeeping tasks.

DYNAMIC DUO

The kidneys are a frequent player in the Cayce readings' discussion of ridding the body of toxic build-up. In tandem, the readings would often discuss the liver which, although it also rightfully belongs as a member of the digestive tract, has a vital and important relationship with the kidneys. Both organs perform important roles in processing and purifying the blood. The liver accomplishes hundreds of important metabolic functions through its processing of your body's life-giving crimson stream. At the same time, the kidneys filter the body's blood several hundred times each day. The readings stress that an imbalance between these two functions can cause the body to toss toxins back into the system rather than eliminate them. And as Chapters 2 and 3 describe, this can result in headache pain.

WATER OF LIFE

The most important rule to follow to keep these organs healthy and thus happy will not come as a surprise. Luckily, it is a simple rule to follow. Drink six to eight glasses of water a day. Intake of an adequate amount of water on a daily basis not only benefits the kidneys and liver, but also the colon and skin as well.

Here's a suggested routine which will help you get into the healthy habit of drinking enough water daily. This routine adds up to an intake of 8 1/2 glasses, giving you some cushion in case you miss a glass or two (but not more) during the day. Notice that the first half glass of water in the morning is warm. Cayce specifically suggested this as an aid to help the digestive system with its eliminations.

When	Count
Upon arising (warm)	1/2
Mid-morning and afternoon	2
Before breakfast, lunch, and dinner	3
After breakfast, lunch, and dinner	3
Total	8 1/2

CASTOR OIL PACKS

One of the most unique and often applied therapies for the elimination system in the Cayce readings involves the use of castor oil. Although many people may think of castor oil as a purgative of the alimentary canal (most often recommended by grandmothers), it has been recognized for centuries as a healing agent for a variety of purposes. In Roman times it was referred to as the *Palma Christi* or palm of Christ. This phrase implies external use, and that's exactly what Cayce suggested.

Specifically, Cayce often recommended a castor oil pack to stimulate the liver. It also has a positive effect upon the gall bladder and colon, can assist lymphatic circulation, dissolve adhesions, reduce inflammation, and improve assimilation within the digestive tract.

A good routine to follow is to apply the pack three consecutive days a week for two to three weeks. Then leave off a week, and resume with another two- to three-week cycle.

Directions for applying a pack can be found in *Appendix D.*

TURPENTINE AND CAMPHOR RUB

For the equivalent stimulation of the kidneys that a castor oil pack provides the liver, the readings suggested a rubbing compound of turpentine, spirits of camphor, and mutton tallow.

Before using this remedy, you should first try a small amount of turpentine on your skin as a test patch to make sure that it does not cause irritation or burning. Once you have established that the turpentine does not have an adverse effect on you, you're ready to begin.

A good routine to follow is to apply this rub two to three consecutive nights during a week you are not using the castor oil packs. You need to experiment with a routine between the pack and the rub that you feel results in better eliminations and higher energy.

SPECIAL TEAS

Herbal teas are becoming more and more common substitutes for caffeine-bearing beverages such as tea and coffee. It's good news, then, that certain teas can also have positive effects upon specific body systems. Two particular teas were recommended to aid the liver and kidneys in their functions.

Watermelon seed tea has long been accepted as an excellent diuretic, containing saltpeter. This tea is found in almost all health food stores. In the summer, however, when watermelons are in season, you can save the seeds (place them in an airtight bag and keep them in a dark place) and use them to make your tea year round. A good way to make watermelon seed tea is to grind the seeds in a food processor when you're ready for a cup of tea. Then fill a tea ball with the grounds and let it steep for several minutes before drinking. You'll find that the tea has a weak color, but don't be discouraged. It can still work wonders for your kidneys!

Ragweed tea is suggested to invigorate the liver and also has a laxative effect upon the colon. Your best bet is to find this tea in a health food store and prepare it using a tea ball. Like all herbs, be sure to store this tea and any others in a dark, dry place so that it will retain its potency.

COLON HEALTH

Your colon, of course, conducts the residue of solid and liquid foods through your body. Keeping it clean and functioning properly increases your body's ability to eliminate its wastes.

As mentioned above, both water and castor oil packs will benefit your colon. Support these with the intake of roughage and natural laxatives as well as colonic irrigations or enemas, and you can keep your colon in superior condition.

Although you will learn a great deal about proper diet in Chapter 6, here's a dietary hint that is of particular benefit to your colon. Get into the habit of eating a raw lunch in the form of a salad or an assortment of raw vegetables. Enjoy a slice of whole grain bread as well. You'll find that your energy is higher all afternoon, and your eliminations will be more regular.

In addition to the fiber of green leafy vegetables and grains, the readings stressed several fruits as natural laxatives, which should be included in the diet, particularly in the mornings and evenings. Stewed figs, raisins, apricots, prunes, and pears were noted as being helpful in this area. As you begin to work with these, notice how your body reacts, and find the best and most helpful way to include them in your diet.

COLON CLEANING

As you know from reading about both tension and migraine headaches, the time will come when you need to flush your system via a colonic or an enema. Cayce stressed that even if your bowels seem regular, there may still be need of hydrotherapy to cleanse the alimentary canal. Specific symptoms, indicating the need for this therapy, might include feelings of heaviness, sleepiness, and dragginess.

(Of course, if such symptoms persist, see your physician.)

Remember, of course, that prevention is always the wiser course than cure. Thus, the readings suggested an inner cleansing on a regular basis. The best way to obtain an inner cleansing is to get a colonic irrigation from a trained professional. Or you can also give yourself an enema at home.

Directions for administering a home enema can be found in *Appendix D.*

BREATHE DEEPLY

It's hard to imagine that your lungs may have something to do with your head. Yet, without your lungs, your head would suffer not only from oxygen loss but from overtoxicity as well. The lungs are one of the lesser recognized organs involved in bodily eliminations. Yet they work regularly through the process of breathing, to release carbon dioxide, the end product of your body's metabolism of oxygen.

Nothing helps your lungs more than fresh air and regular, deep respirations. First and foremost, you should observe your breathing patterns. Do you use your diaphragm and breathe with depth and regularity? Breathing is probably one of the body's functions most taken for granted. Become conscious of your respirations and take steps to improve the "exercise" you give your lungs.

You'll find many positive suggestions for giving your lungs a workout in the exercise section of Chapter 6. In short, whenever you exercise, be sure to take deep, regular breaths as an important part of the process.

Another suggestion is to pause several times during the day, especially when you find yourself in a fresh-air environment, and breathe in deeply and out forcefully. This helps expand your lungs and jog loose toxic particles trapped in the recesses of your lungs and nasal passages. In addition, deep, slow breaths can help your body relax, releasing mental and physical strain.

A final word. If you happen to smoke, you should consider discontinuing as a measure to improve your current health and increase your longevity. Enough has been said in recent years in the media to indicate the health hazards of both primary and secondary smoke. Aside from the risks the chemicals in cigarettes pose, there is the reduced capacity of your lungs to take in oxygen and eliminate toxins. Give this thought some consideration as you try to launch a healthier life style.

SURPRISE APPEARANCE

Finally, the least noticed organ of elimination is actually seldom recognized as an organ at all! Your skin is, in fact, your body's largest organ and one of its most vital. This protective organ covers seventeen square feet on the average adult. Not only does it eliminate fluids and toxins, it also protects your inner organs and helps regulate your body's temperature. So you can see its oft overlooked importance.

Supplying your body with ample water is the first step toward aiding the skin in toxin elimination. Why? Because water is the agent, in the form of perspiration, by which the skin eliminates wastes. Refer to the chart on page 38 which outlines a program for insuring that your daily intake of water is adequate.

There are three additional practices that will be of benefit to both your skin and circulation. They are hot baths, steam therapy, and massages. All are highly enjoyable and beneficial. Here's a word about the benefits of taking the time to relax with a hot bath or steam. (We'll cover the value of regular massages in the context of circulation.)

A nice, relaxing hot bath is often one of the victims of our rushed and hectic life styles. Jumping in the shower and out again three or four minutes later serves simply to cleanse, not relax. As a part of your new health-creating life style consider including taking a long, hot bath now and then to relax. Supplement your bath with a firm rubdown of peanut oil either before or after you hop in the tub (*before* if you have to dress and go somewhere later; *after* if you can put on your pajamas and robe). The hot bath will open up your pores and promote perspiration, which will help release toxins from your body. The oil rubdown will condition and stimulate your skin (and circulation).

A steam serves the same purposes as a hot, relaxing bath, though it will generate more perspiration and give your pores an even deeper workout. You can give yourself a home steam by following the directions in *Appendix D.*

GETTING CIRCULATED

As mentioned earlier, your body has two major circulatory systems: the arteriovenous system and the lymphatic system. These two work as a team. The blood carries and delivers nutrients to each and every cell of your body; the lymph removes the wastes which result as cells absorb and burn the energy they derive from the nutrients. In short, the blood brings in the groceries, the lymph takes out the trash.

You're probably familiar with the workings of your arterial circulation. The heart provides the pressure necessary to keep the blood coursing through your arteries. It is a well-designed pump which is fully capable, if in good health, to accomplish its purpose. Exercise, massage, and a heart-healthful diet are excellent ways to keep it in tiptop shape for peak performance.

You're probably less familiar with the structure and functioning of your lymphatic circulation. First, to give you a visual idea of what your lymph is, think about the last time you cut yourself. Did you notice that not only did you bleed, but your body also seemed to bring a clear fluid to the scene of the wound? That fluid is your lymph. It is just as plentiful in your body as is your blood.

Not only does it differ in function from your blood, the lymph differs in one other significant way. It does not have a well-primed pump to provide the pressure necessary to move it throughout your body. Rather, it relies on the pressure caused by the flexing and movement of muscles in your daily activities, the most important of which is the diaphragm. Thus, exercise, massage, and proper breathing—all of which stimulate muscle activity—are important therapies to maximize the effectiveness of your lymphatic circulation.

You'll find specific advice on exercise in Chapter 6.

MASSAGE

Getting a massage on a regular basis is as important to our health as diet or exercise. Not only does it have a calming effect on an emotional level, it also stimulates the blood and lymph circulation, enabling them to perform their life-giving functions. The best way to take advantage of the therapeutic effects of massage is to find a professional massage therapist who provides you with a massage that *you* feel is of benefit to you. Try to establish a regular day and time, preferably once a week, for your massage. Then, stick with it. The benefits will be immeasurable.

The reality may be, however, that you cannot find a good massage therapist or the time to visit one regularly. Another way to take advantage of massage is to administer a self-massage. This practice will help you get in touch with your body, which will in turn promote better health. Combine a thorough self-massage with your hot-bath routine for excellent results.

General guidelines for doing so can be found in *Appendix D.*

Chapter 5

HEADACHE-PREVENTION DIET

HOW DIET HELPS

You're about to learn some diet basics which will promote good health and some diet specifics which will help prevent and cure headache pain. The general principle behind the acid/alkaline-balanced diet included here was suggested to many people suffering from headaches—and people suffering from tinnitus as well.

First, you need to know that fueling your body for optimum health involves a great deal more than just the foods you eat. What you consume—your diet—is simply the first step toward providing your body with the energy it needs to carry on its duties. Assimilation, the second step, determines how effectively your body absorbs the nutrients which are in your food. The final step is the value you derive from your food intake. This all-important aspect of eating called nutrition is determined both by what you eat and by how that food reacts chemically within your body.

Why are diet, assimilation, and nutrition important? Cayce observed that the body is in a constant state of growth and restoration, long after the formative years. In fact, he indicated that the body has the capacity to regenerate itself every seven years. This restoration happens at the cellular level, as three to eight billion cells die on a daily basis and are replaced by newly formed cells. It is important, then, that we provide our bodies with the fuel necessary for this important growth and renewal process.

FRAME OF MIND

Your frame of mind is a very important, though seemingly intangible, part of your diet. To get the proper nutrition from the foods you eat, it is important to take time to eat slowly. Doing so allows the digestive juices (beginning with the saliva in the mouth) to adequately break down the food you eat for proper nutrition. Bolting food can cause your body to consume extra energy to digest it—thus robbing other bodily systems of much needed energy. Therefore, remember to chew your food thoroughly as the first step toward reaping the benefits of your diet.

Here's another common-sense hint. Never eat when you're worried or upset. If you've ever made the mistake of eating after a stressful meeting at work or on the heels of an argument with a loved one, you may well know firsthand the wisdom of this suggestion.

Finally, Cayce added that it is just as detrimental to your health to eat simply to pass the time of day. You must eat with a purpose—that of giving your body life so that you can better be of service in the world. Thus the food you eat becomes food for the spirit as well as food for the body. Abstract though this may seem, remember how important your *spirit* is to your health. Keeping your spirit healthy by being kind to your body—and kind to others with the labors of your body—is an important part of your diet plan.

EAT THE RIGHT THING

An equally important factor in proper diet, of course, deals with *what food you eat* and in *what combinations*.

You must be mindful of whether the foods you eat create an acid or alkaline state within your body. The acid/alkaline balance of your body is a major factor influencing your health as well as the strength of your immune system. Specifically, Cayce indicated that overacidity can make the system prone to headaches.

The natural acid/alkaline state or pH of the body is 7.4 (slightly alkaline); on this scale 7 is neutral, below 7 is more acid; and above 7 more alkaline. Although the blood usually remains almost constant at 7.4, other body fluids can fluctuate. It's your job to keep tabs on your acid/alkaline balance—and take corrective measures if possible. The best way to regulate your acid/alkaline balance is by diet. The outline below will tell you how this can be accomplished.

Appendix D offers you instructions for testing your acid/alkaline balance.

THE RIGHT FOODS

Alkaline-Forming Foods
(Optimally 80% of Your Diet)

All fruits except cranberries, plums, and prunes

All vegetables except for lentils and corn

All milk including buttermilk

Almonds, brazil nuts, chestnuts, coconut, hazelnuts

Coffee, tea, molasses, brown sugar, brewer's yeast

Acid-Forming Foods
(Optimally 20% of Your Diet)

All meats except for mincemeat

All cereals and bakery products except for soybeans

All cheeses and eggs

Peanuts, pecans, walnuts

It's also important to eat the right foods in the correct combinations to maintain a balanced system. An added bonus in properly combining foods is the nutrition you can derive from them. Remember, nutrition results from the chemical breakdown of foods within your body. How you combine your foods is critical to how they react within your body. The practice of eating the right foods together can have an immense impact upon the success of your diet and the future of your health. Why? Different foods require different responses from your body to get maximal digestion. Poorly combining foods can create incomplete digestion and toxins which tax your eliminations. As you've learned, poor digestion can prompt headache pain.

THE RIGHT COMBINATIONS

The following combinations of foods were suggested by Cayce as being particularly beneficial:

At least three vegetables that grow above the ground for each that grows below the ground

Gelatin with fruits and vegetables to help absorb nutrients

Figs, dates, and cornmeal

Small amounts of lemon or lime juice with orange or grapefruit juices

These combinations were mentioned as being detrimental to your general health:

Milk at the same meal as citrus fruits and juices

Cereals at the same meal as citrus fruits and juices

Coffee with milk or cream

Raw apples eaten at the same time as other foods

Two or more starches at the same meal

Sugary foods with starches

Meats and cheeses with starches

SOME SPECIAL DIET TIPS

Below are some special foods and diet tips that the headache-wary person should include in the diet. They may seem like odd suggestions at first—but remember that many natural remedies are just as surprising in their benefits as they are in their content!

WATER, WATER, WATER

As you learned in Chapter 4, water is vital to health. Be sure to consume six to eight glasses of water a day. If you are not currently including this amount of water (or near to it), then it is probably the single most important dietary change you can make. Don't shortcut yourself on this helpful hint and you'll reap the benefits in increased energy and renewed vigor.

BEEF JUICE

Beef juice helps build the blood without introducing excess amounts of fat into your system. Since general fatigue and debilitation were often mentioned as causes of headaches, this remedy is one you should take seriously. Iron is, after all, a necessary mineral for bodily strength and energy. Preparation of beef juice is really very simple. To begin, gather these items:

1/4 lb. of raw, lean beef

32 oz. empty glass jar with top

Large sauce pan

Small wash cloth

Place wash cloth in the bottom of the sauce pan (this will prevent jar from breaking or cracking). Cut beef into one-inch cubes and place in jar. Cover with top very loosely. Place jar on top of cloth in pan. Fill sauce pan with enough water to come half way up the side of the glass jar. Bring water to a boil. Then, simmer for two to three hours, adding water to pan as necessary.

When done, remove from heat and let jar and contents cool. Then, squeeze excess juice from meat into the jar. Discard meat. Refrigerate, but do not keep it longer than three days. Sip it two to four times a day, no more than a tablespoon at a time.

GELATIN

Pure gelatin was mentioned by Cayce numerous times as a food supplement that helped the body assimilate the nutrients in other foods. It was particularly suggested in combination with fruits and vegetables. A good way to take advantage of this "miracle substance" is to combine it in congealed vegetable and fruit salads. Some people mix it in their fruit and vegetable juices as well. This is one remedy which can be as tasty as your imagination (or cookbook) allows it to be—and beneficial to your head and health as well.

TYPICAL MENU

The following menu gives you an idea of the general approach you should take to your diet. Three meals a day is an important part of the food formula—helping your body maintain a regular level of nutritional intake. Cayce prefaced this menu with a statement indicating that it is simply a guideline to be considered. There are dozens of variations within these suggestions, allowing you to enjoy a varied and interesting diet.

Mornings. Have either a dry, high fiber cereal, a hot grain cereal, *or* citrus fruit whole or as juice. If you enjoy toast, dark-bread toast such as pumpernickel, rye or whole wheat is best. You may have a moderate amount of coffee but Cayce warned against having cream with it, indicating that this combination was a stress upon the heart and the digestive system.

Noon. Raw vegetables, as fresh as possible. Especially carrots, celery, lettuce, and any other green vegetable. Vegetable soup is a good option for a cold day. Pure, fresh carrot juice, even in as small a quantity as an ounce, is an excellent supplement to this meal. A piece or two of whole wheat bread rounds out your noon meal with added nutritive value.

Dinner. A little meat if desired, preferably fish, fowl, or lamb. Include shell fish, high in iodine content and thus good for your thyroid. Include an abundance of cooked vegetables, eliminating potatoes. Yams can be enjoyed occasionally.

Chapter 6

ATTITUDE ADJUSTERS

STRESS AND HEADACHES

You've learned a lot about your body and how its internal systems can affect your head. But there's a multitude of ways your head can affect your head as well! Anger, worry, resentment—all of those emotions which not only cause stress but *are* stress in and of themselves—can wear down your mind and thinking processes. The result is often fatigue and sometimes headaches. Fifty to seventy percent of migraine sufferers mention emotional factors as being the most important for triggering their headaches. Below are three ways to help you begin to lessen the stress in your life—meditation, pre-sleep suggestions, and exercise.

THE STRESS REDUCER

Meditation is a number-one stress reducer which has an added benefit. Not only does it help relax you by taking you away from the stresses of everyday life—it also gets you in tune with the divine wisdom within. As you may remember, this wisdom is a key ingredient in your health and wholeness.

Here are the main elements important in meditation. You may be surprised at how simple they are. Practice them with consistency, and you'll soon begin to feel the results.

Set a Regular Time As you have probably learned in your own life, human beings are creatures of habit. Setting a regular time for any activity, whether it be an evening walk or a morning break, makes it much more likely that you will indeed undertake that activity. Meditation is no exception. Set a regular time for meditation, allowing 15-20 minutes for starters, and you will find it easier to actually devote time to this important process. Also, you will discover that settling into the routine of meditation allows you to quiet and focus your thoughts more easily. It is as though your mind gets in the habit of a quiet time and thus slips into the meditative state with greater ease.

Learn to Relax If you could learn to relax on a regular basis, your health would improve immeasurably. One of the simplest benefits of regular meditation is that you find a small amount of time daily to relax body, mind, and soul. You also learn what it feels like for your body to relax—a feeling you can come back to at other times during the day. And believe it or not, no matter how hectic may be the day which looms ahead or spirals behind, relaxation can be yours with relative ease.

Here are some powerful relaxers to consider:

Light stretching. Just prior to meditation take a moment to stretch your body by simply reaching upward, straightening your spine. Do whatever stretching motions feel good to you, feeling the release of tension in your muscles.

Head and neck exercise. A specific exercise which is especially helpful prior to meditation is the head and neck exercise, which is described in detail on pages 64 and 65. This exercise releases tension and increases circulation to the head and neck area.

Soothing music. Gentle music can provide a special nourishment to the soul. Playing peaceful and calming music in the background during meditation can help your mind release the cares of the day and thus focus more adeptly during the meditative process.

Reading inspirational or spiritual verse. Another quieting activity is to select a book, perhaps the Bible or a special book of poetry, to read for a moment as you settle down to meditate. Let your mind focus on the positive images and thoughts as you read.

Breathing. Special breathing techniques can be a tremendous relaxation aid. Here's a simple one with which to begin. As you relax, breathe in deeply, visualizing peace and calm flowing in as you breathe. Then breathe out deeply, releasing any tension and stress you might have as you exhale. Continue this technique until you begin to feel more tranquil.

Sit or Lie with Your Spine Straight It is important

to assume a position with your spine as straight as possible. This allows for the best flow of nerve impulses along your spinal cord and throughout your body. You may choose to sit in a straight-backed chair, assume the lotus position, or even lie flat on your back. In the event you are sitting, place your hands, open and relaxed, in your lap. If you are lying on your back, join your hands over your abdominal area.

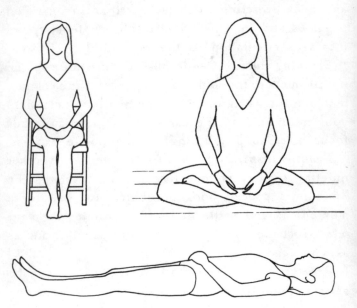

Begin with Prayer Begin your meditation time with a few moments of prayer. In your prayer, remember to be open to God's will. During this time, try to establish a sense of peace and calm within yourself, and a sense of openness and desire to be of service. Once you have quieted yourself, it is time to begin meditating.

A special note is important here. If you are unable to become peaceful within, perhaps because you are anxious or upset about something in your life, remain in a prayerful state. Attempting to meditate while feeling negative emotions can stir up those feelings to an even greater extent. Later, when you feel in a calmer state, then you may attempt to meditate.

Work with a Special Affirmation An affirmation or inspirational phrase is an important element of meditation. It may be one of your favorite Bible passages or a verse from an inspiring poem. Whatever phrase you choose, it should encompass your highest ideals and principles. Use this phrase as a focal point for your experience. You will probably want to change your affirmation from time to time. It is wise, however, to use the same one for a week or two at a time, so that you become familiar with it. Just like selecting a specific time for meditation, using a familiar affirmation helps make your meditation period more successful. We are, after all, better at what we practice at!

Experience the Silence After your prayer, begin to repeat your affirmation quietly, but aloud. Try to feel and experience the *meaning* or *spirit* of the words. The feelings your affirmation creates should begin to make you feel uplifted and at greater peace. When you feel that you have raised your consciousness above your ordinary state, become quiet and focus upon the feeling or spirit the affirmation has created. Hold this spirit for as long as you are able.

Deal Positively with Distractions It is quite natural to become distracted by other thoughts as you meditate. When this occurs, do not be discouraged and quit. Ask for a blessing upon whatever has distracted you and begin to repeat your affirmation again. You may choose to simply think about the words of the affirmation at this point, rather than speaking them aloud. Once you have captured their spirit again and feel more elevated, stop thinking about the specific words once again. Simply focus upon the inner silence you have created. This inner silence is the essence of meditation. In this silence you encounter the spirit, love, and wisdom of God.

Close with a Prayer for Others During meditation you have tapped into a spiritual energy which must be dispersed as you conclude your meditation period. Do so by closing your meditation with a prayer for others. This selfless act will complete your quiet time in a positive way.

SUMMING UP MEDITATION

Meditation and prayer were vital ingredients in Cayce's approach to life. Through this kind of attunement to the spirit, Cayce indicated that therapies applied "externally, internally, through the diet, through all portions of the activities, may bring coordination, cooperation in the physical forces of the body." (1211-2) So, take the time. It will be an important element in your journey to heal your head and improve your health.

POWER OF THE SUBCONSCIOUS MIND

The subconscious mind is a powerful ally in your quest for health and wholeness. As we discussed earlier, the subconscious mind directs much of the activity of the autonomic nervous system. This is the system sending signals to the farthest outposts of your body, signals which can either bring health or illness. Meditation will help you align your mental and spiritual bodies with the Spirit. Pre-sleep suggestions and visualization will be further aids in materializing the wisdom of the spirit, through the mind, to the body.

PRE-SLEEP SUGGESTION

The Cayce readings suggested a powerful, useful, and effective method for implanting positive, constructive thoughts in the subconscious to help bring about positive change. Just prior to going to sleep, the readings indicated that the subconscious mind is most accessible. The use of "pre-sleep" suggestion can gently persuade your mind to construct a foundation of positive thoughts upon which to build your new life style.

To harness the power of pre-sleep suggestion to help overcome headache pain, you'll want to make your own pre-sleep tape. Making this tape is actually quite easy. Begin by reading through the following script to become familiar with it. Feel free to modify it to make it more personalized to you. Follow only one rule in making any minor changes—make sure that the words or phrases you substitute are positive and uplifting. Once you are comfortable with your script, sit down with a tape recorder and record, using a soothing, slowly paced voice, and pausing comfortably between phrases (indicated by " . . . "). You might like to have relaxing music playing in the background so that it is a backdrop to your voice. This tape of affirmations will help program your subconscious to develop positive mental attitudes and patterns about healing.

You will gain the optimum benefit from this tape by listening to it on a nightly basis just as you are going to sleep. For best results play the tape at a soft and comfortable volume near your bedside. If you have a cassette player that will play both sides consecutively, you may want to record the script on each side so that it can play twice as long without interruption. Most important, set the tape up so that it turns off automatically.

PRE-SLEEP TAPE SCRIPT
(to be read aloud onto cassette tape)

Consider lying down now . . . closing your eyes . . . and relaxing. Feel yourself gently drifting off into the peacefulness of sleep . . . feel yourself resting . . . and relaxing . . . focus on your breathing, how it is bringing peace and relaxation with every breath . . . and deeper relaxation . . . feel the relaxation that your steady, deep breathing brings to your body . . . notice how your muscles are relaxing . . . first your feet feel the lightness of relaxation . . . with every muscle loosening and relaxing . . . now your lower legs, feeling the pleasure of relaxation, becoming lighter and looser with each deep breath . . . feel how your breath travels through your legs and thighs bringing relaxation to your lower body . . . allow the waves of calm and peace to travel from your legs upward into your buttocks . . . your waist and your trunk . . . your muscles are becoming harmonious with one another . . . bringing one another a feeling of deep, deep relaxation . . . so relaxed that your body is feeling lighter and lighter . . . your fingers and hands are relaxing . . . with each breath they are relaxing and responding to the sense of peace you are feeling . . . your arms . . . your shoulders . . . feel how they are relaxing . . . with each breath they are relaxing . . . and sinking into the comfort of sleep and deep relaxation . . . feel how your shoulders and neck are settling into a state of relaxation . . . loosening with each breath . . . loosening with each breath . . . now your neck and head are feeling light . . . and relaxed . . . and you're pleasantly drowsy . . . drifting into a pleasant . . . peaceful . . . sleep . . . awaken to the healing of the spirit . . . flowing freely through the lightness of your body . . . you are open to the healing touch of the spirit . . . to the wisdom of the spirit that makes you whole and harmonious . . . you are allowing this healing spirit to inspire you . . . you see yourself working in harmony with this spirit . . . you are at one with the wise healer within . . . doing your part to give your body the nourishment it needs to heal . . . you are eating health-giving foods . . . you are allowing their nourishment to regulate your body in all that it does as it helps you feel better . . . your body is your friend . . . and you are helping it align with the spirit within to be strong and whole and healthy

63

. . . you are drifting into a natural, comfortable sleep
. . . a place where you are safe and at peace
. . . you are being carried off into a healing and
rejuvenating sleep . . . where you are relaxed
. . . and being healed . . . you are being carried
off into sleep . . . where you are relaxed . . . and
being healed . . . feel the waves of calm and peace
as they caress and nurture your body . . .

THE EXERCISE INVESTMENT

Harold J. Reilly, prominent physical therapist and
author of *The Edgar Cayce Handbook for Health
Through Drugless Therapy*, once said that the best
exercises are the ones that you do! This humorous
statement is full of simple wisdom. How many people
do you know who talk about exercising but do not
follow their routines with consistency? We've all been
in that same, lurching boat at some time in our
lives. For a week, maybe two, we go about exercising
with great energy and determination. But so often
time pressures, gradual lack of interest, or even a
pulled muscle from overdoing halt what progress
we've made. Regardless of the vigor of our occasional
work-outs, they are not as beneficial as moderate,
consistent, and persistent exercise.

HEAD AND NECK

A unique exercise for the head and neck was
mentioned in the Cayce readings over 300 times.
It was primarily mentioned for eye and ear problems—
both of which can complicate matters in your head.

Sit with your spine erect and your shoulders relaxed. Bend your head forward three times, backward three times, to the right three times, to the left three times. Then, gently rotate your head 360 degrees in both directions three times. Do this series slowly and deliberately.

This exercise brings more circulation to the head and neck. Improved eyesight, more acute hearing, and greater relaxation are but a few of the many benefits of this routine.

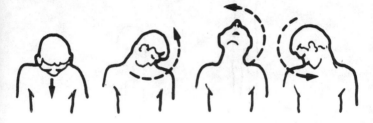

MORNING WAKE-UP

A good exercise for the morning is to stand straight and tall, preferably in front of an open window (if the air outside is fresh and clean). Gradually rise up on your tiptoes, inhaling slowly and deeply, and gently bring your arms upward over your head. Then, bend forward and bring your fingertips down to touch your toes. Just as your hands reach the floor, exhale in a single, forceful breath. If you are newly beginning this exercise routine, repeat this exercise three times. If you feel that you can comfortably do more, work up to ten repetitions.

This stretching exercise is particularly good at giving your respiratory system a morning wake-up. An added bonus is that the tightening of the leg muscles and employment of the diaphragm are particularly effective in moving the lymph, which has slowed down a great deal during your night's rest.

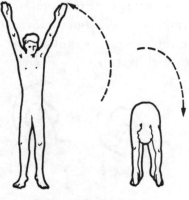

PELVIC ROLL

A specific evening exercise often recommended is the pelvic roll. Position yourself on the floor, face down, as if preparing to do a push-up, but place your feet flush against a wall. Raise yourself up on your arms, then rotate your hips in a circle—three times clockwise, three times counterclockwise. If you find this position too strenuous, you may actually rest on your elbows rather than your hands when assuming the push-up position.

Cayce indicated that this exercise, which rotates the lower portions of the body, would help alter circulation in a way that aided in better assimilation and eliminations.

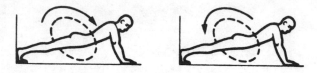

WALKING

Cayce recommended walking as a general exercise which would benefit everyone. A brisk walk accomplishes several goals. It exercises muscles which helps stimulate your arterial and venous circulation. An added bonus is that it also stimulates lymph flow, thereby helping move toxins on to the organs of elimination. Breathe in fresh air as you walk and your lungs will benefit; build up a light sweat and your skin will be cleansed as well.

The ideal routine is to take a walk in the morning after breakfast, and one again in the evening a half-hour or so after a light, nutritious meal. Swing your arms as you walk and breathe deeply. You may find, of course, that one walk a day is all that you can comfortably work into your schedule. Pick the time that is the least hectic for you so that your walk can be peaceful and calm. Enjoy.

CONCLUSION

It is hoped that this book has taught you some unique and useful tips on head and neck pain, tips you can bring to your aid when planning a strategy to overcome your aches and pains—whether they be frequent or periodic. Admittedly, some of the suggestions may seem a bit out of the ordinary. Who would have believed that digestive problems could come to rest in your head? Or, that a problem in your spine could interrupt your entire body's communication systems to the point that muscles in your head and neck tense up? Strange though these suggestions may be, many people have found them to be helpful in the treatment of headaches. We hope you will soon be among the ranks of the victorious.

But don't just wait until your headaches become so distressing that you have to wage war on them to win. Try to stay ahead of the game. If you suffer only from periodic headaches, don't allow yourself to become complacent about your health. Take the suggestions in this book seriously, and ward off future head and neck pain. In the process, you'll find that your general health will improve—and possibly your state of mind.

The fact is that in today's hectic world, we are all threatened by the ill effects of stress. And poor diet. And unhealthy health practices. It's not as easy to stay healthy, nor is it as easy to get well. Unless, of course, you begin now to awaken your body to the healer within. That way, when you need this healer as a friend, you'll already be familiar and in touch with its miraculous powers. And true health will be yours for the asking.

APPENDIX A

WHO WAS EDGAR CAYCE?

Edgar Cayce exhibited unusual psychic ability at an early age and soon became known for his remarkable clairvoyant gifts. In a self-induced hypnotic state, he was able to diagnose illnesses and prescribe remedies with remarkable success. Often referred to as "the sleeping prophet" and the world's most documented psychic, Edgar Cayce left behind a legacy of over 14,000 psychic readings covering such subjects as healing, dreams, meditation, reincarnation, prophecy, and psychic ability.

Born in 1877 in Hopkinsville, Kentucky, he discovered by accident that he could absorb information on any particular subject merely by napping for a while on a book pertaining to that topic. At the age of fifteen he suffered an accident and, while in a coma, instructed his astonished parents to prepare a poultice to be applied at the base of his brain. The application fully restored him.

After he reached adulthood, his job as a salesman was threatened by a mysterious paralysis of the throat muscles which medical doctors were unable to treat. He consulted a hypnotist, and it was under the subsequent trance that Edgar correctly diagnosed his condition and prescribed an almost immediate cure.

Not long after, Edgar discovered that his gift could be used to help others, and what followed was over forty years of helping people from his self-induced state of unconsciousness. For twenty-two of these years, his readings were largely confined to medical problems; however, the scope of Edgar's abilities expanded in later years to include such subjects as meditation, dreams, reincarnation, and the Bible.

Edgar Cayce is regarded today as one of the most significant explorers of the human psyche in the twentieth century.

APPENDIX B

HOW THE A.R.E. CAN HELP YOU

A wealth of information from the Edgar Cayce readings is available to you on hundreds of topics, from astrology and arthritis to universal laws and world affairs, through the organization which Edgar Cayce founded in 1931, the Association for Research and Enlightenment, Inc.

The facilities and benefits offered by the A.R.E. include the largest body of documented psychic information anywhere in the world: the 14,263 Cayce readings, copies of which are housed in the A.R.E. Library/Conference Center in Virginia Beach, Virginia. These readings have been indexed under 10,000 different topics and are currently being placed on computer. They are available to the public.

Membership in the A.R.E. is inexpensive and includes benefits such as: the bimonthly magazine, *Venture Inward;* home-study lessons in spiritual awareness and growth; the A.R.E. Library, available to you through book borrowing by mail, offering collections of the actual Edgar Cayce readings as well as access to one of the world's best parapsychological book collections; and the names of medical doctors or health care professionals in your area who are willing to work with the remedies prescribed in the Edgar Cayce readings.

As an organization on the leading edge of exciting new fields of study, A.R.E. also presents seminars around the nation, led by prominent authorities in various fields and exploring such areas as parapsychology, dreams, meditation, personal growth, world religions, reincarnation and life after death, and holistic health.

The unique path to personal growth outlined in the Cayce readings is developed through a worldwide program of study groups. These informal groups meet weekly in private homes—right in your community—for friendly consciousness-expanding discussions.

A.R.E. maintains a visitors' center that offers a well-stocked bookstore, exhibits, classes, a movie, and audiovisual presentations to introduce seekers from all walks of life to the fascinating concepts found in the Cayce readings.

A.R.E. conducts ongoing research into the helpfulness of both the medical and nonmedical readings, often giving members the opportunity to participate in the studies themselves.

For more information and a free color brochure, write or phone:

A.R.E.

P.O. Box 595

67th Street and Atlantic Avenue

Virginia Beach, VA 23451-0595; (804) 428-3588

APPENDIX C

WHERE TO FIND THE REMEDIES AND INGREDIENTS

Some of the formulations mentioned in the Edgar Cayce readings are available from:

Home Health Products
P.O. Box 3130
Virginia Beach, VA 23454

Information about the Impedance Device is available from:

The A.R.E. Clinic
4018 N. 40th St.
Phoenix, AZ 85018

APPENDIX D

DIRECTIONS FOR SELF-ADMINISTERED THERAPIES

Below are directions for the preparation and application of several home therapies which will help you prevent and control head and neck pain. This medicine chest of remedies is for your convenient reference. The benefits of these therapies are described in the main portion of this book.

As with any therapy, it is ideal to understand the benefit it is having to your body. The therapy is more effective if you can focus on its purpose as you apply it and visualize it having the desired effect. Each therapy below includes a page reference you can flip to in order to refresh your understanding of its healing benefits.

Acid/Alkaline Balance

Refer to Chapter 5, pages 49 and 50.

The best way to test your acid-alkaline balance is by using nitrazine paper (found at most drug stores) to determine the pH of your saliva. It is ideal to perform this test in the morning before eating or drinking. Take a paper strip and wet it with your saliva. Read the instructions on the package to determine your exact range on the pH scale. Remember, you're aiming for a slightly alkaline system (pH 7 or higher), and diet is the best way to achieve it. So, if you test acid, review your diet and make changes to bring your system into better balance.

Enema

Refer to Chapter 4, pages 41 and 42.

Here are some basic guidelines for a home enema. First, gather the following items:

Enema bag

Vaseline

Isopropyl alcohol

Pure spring water

Two large towels

Plastic trash bag

Salt 1 tsp.

Glyco-Thymoline 1 tsp.

Sodium bicarbonate 1 tsp.

Begin by sterilizing the tube or nozzle of the enema bag by soaking it in alcohol or boiling water. Then, rinse it thoroughly. Prepare a quart of lukewarm spring water (98.6° F.), adding a teaspoon each of sodium bicarbonate and salt. Spread out a large plastic trash bag beneath several towels on the bed or floor and lie down on your left side. Have the bag elevated above the level of your body. Coat the enema nozzle with Vaseline and insert it two to four inches into your rectum. (Caution: do not force it.) Allow one-third of the water to enter your colon slowly. If you begin to cramp, clamp the tube shut and take several deep breaths. Then continue once the cramps subside. Once one-third of the water is inside, turn over on your back and allow the next third to enter, following the same procedure. Finally, shift to your right side and empty the remaining fluid from the bag into your body.

Now, try to hold the solution for five to fifteen minutes, moving gently to swish the fluid around in the colon. This allows the fluid to soften and loosen the wastes. Your next step is the bathroom, where you can now expel the water.

Rest a few moments, then repeat the process until the fluid which leaves your body is mostly clear. Administer a final round of water, adding a teaspoon of Glyco-Thymoline (which you can find in your health food store) to the water (instead of the salt and soda) to serve as an antiseptic to the colon area.

Castor Oil Pack

Refer to Chapter 4, pages 38 and 39.

For preparing and applying a castor oil pack, gather these items:

Cold-pressed castor oil

2' square of wool or cotton flannel

Large towel

Two safety pins

Small plastic trash bag

Electric heating pad

Glass or ceramic bowl

Glass jar or plastic container

2 tsp. baking soda added to a container with 1 quart of warm water

Pour heated castor oil into glass or ceramic bowl. Fold the flannel cloth four times to form a 1' square. Place it in the bowl, saturating it with oil. Wring out the excess. Now position the pack slightly to the right on your abdomen, over the liver. Cover the pack with the plastic bag, put the heating pad on top of it, and place a towel on top of these layers, wrapping it around the body and fastening it with safety pins. Then, turn on the heating pad. You may want to lie on a plastic bag or towel to protect the bed sheets.

A good routine is to apply the pack for one-hour periods in the evening three days in a row for three weeks. Leave off a week, and repeat the three-day/three-week cycle, using the same days of the week and times as before. (Women should not apply the pack during their menstrual cycle.) Store the pack in a glass jar or plastic container. Packs may be reused any number of times, but should not be used by another individual.

Dip a rag into the warm water with the baking soda and clean the abdomen. The oil will contain toxins brought out through the skin and, if the abdomen is not properly cleansed, these toxins may be reabsorbed.

Home Steam

Refer to Chapter 4, pages 44 and 45.

Here are the directions for setting up a homemade steam cabinet. Begin by gathering the following items:

Straight-backed wooden chair

Two towels

Hot plate

Pan of water to boil

Oil or ingredient for steam additive

Old sheet

Thermometer

Pie rack

Custard cup

Find a straight-backed chair, preferably wooden, which will not be damaged by short-term heat and moisture. Drape the chair in towels so that you won't burn your body or the backs of your legs. Place a hot plate and pan of boiling water beneath the chair. Find an old sheet that you'll use as your "steam sheet" again and again. Cut a hole in the middle of the sheet large enough to fit your head through.

Just prior to your steam, drink three glasses of water. Now, undress and sit on the chair, draping the sheet around you like a tent. Be sure that the sheet does not come in contact with the hot plate. Wrap a towel around your neck to keep the steam from escaping.

For safety's sake, have a friend or family member nearby who can check on you and provide you with drinking water to keep your body fluids balanced and to increase perspiration. Be sure to check your pulse and temperature periodically. Your pulse rate should remain below 140 beats per minute and your temperature below 104° F.

When you have worked up a good sweat, stand up slowly, check to see that you're not feeling faint, and proceed to the bathroom. Take a cleansing shower, and afterward rub your body firmly with peanut oil, massaging your muscles and joints with deep, even strokes.

Now that you know how to prepare a home steam cabinet, you may want to add special healing substances and oils to the steam process to aid in stimulating eliminations. Common additives are Atomidine, witch hazel, pine oil, wintergreen, lavender, tincture of myrrh, benzoin, and eucalyptus oil.

Find a small oven-proof glass dish or ceramic container (like a custard cup) and add a teaspoon of your choice of healing ingredient (only one type in any given steam). Float this in the pan of boiling water or place it over the water on a pie rack. The substance will vaporize as a result of the heat and help stimulate the skin.

Turpentine and Camphor Rub

Refer to Chapter 4, page 39.

For preparing and applying a turpentine and camphor rub, gather the following items:

2 oz. mutton tallow

2 oz. turpentine

2 oz. camphor

Melt the mutton tallow. Then allow it to cool, but before it congeals add the turpentine and camphor, pouring the ingredients down the inside wall of the pan to avoid a spattering. Stir together and store in a brown container with name and date of preparation. You can keep this compound up to one year.

Rub on lower back over the kidneys. Cover with two thicknesses of cotton flannel to increase effectiveness. Also, consider applying a heating pad to help your body absorb the healing compound.

Remember to test the turpentine on a patch of skin before applying it to make sure a skin irritation does not result.

Impedance Device

Refer to Chapter 3, page 26.

The Radio-Active Appliance, also known as the Impedance Device, helps energize and balance the subtle electric energies which are vital forces within the body. Specifically, Cayce indicated that the device helps balance the flow of blood and nerves. Thus, the positive effect the device can have in the treatment of headaches is obvious.

Cayce's readings gave specific instructions for building this device. Though you'll want to refer to *Appendix C* to find out where to obtain this device, the following information gives you an understanding of the device and how it is used.

The design of the device is similar to that of a leaky capacitor. Basically it is a sealed copper can which contains two pieces of carbon steel with pieces of glass in between. The can is filled with charcoal which surrounds the carbon steel and glass dividers. At the top of the can, extending from the tops of the two pieces of carbon steel, are connectors, one black and one red, to which are attached copper wires with nickel electrodes at the end.

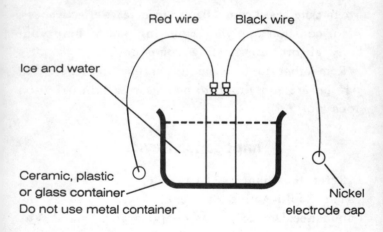

To use this device, you work in cycles. On each day, it is first necessary to "charge" the device by placing it in a glass or ceramic container of ice water for thirty minutes. Then, attach the wires in the following manner:

Day One	black wire to right wrist and red wire to left ankle
Day Two	black wire to left wrist and red wire to right ankle
Day Three	red wire to right wrist and black wire to left ankle
Day Four	red wire to left wrist and black wire to right ankle

Apply this therapy for forty minutes to an hour every evening to complete an entire cycle of four days. Then leave off for a period of time and begin again. Use the time you're applying the Impedance Device to meditate and relax. This will help speed your healing process along the way.

Self-Massage

Refer to Chapter 4, page 46.

You can effectively massage many parts of your body. Below are some basic rules to keep in mind as well as a suggested order for your massage:

Oils

1) Peanut oil is excellent for massage and is particularly beneficial for nerves, muscles, skin, and joints.

2) Olive oil is particularly good for the muscles and stimulates mucous-membrane activity.

3) The following oil mixture combines the healing benefits of the above basic oils. Begin with the peanut

oil as the base and add the rest of the ingredients in order. Shake well before use.

6 oz. peanut oil

2 oz. olive oil

2 oz. rose water

1 tbsp. dissolved lanolin

General Guidelines

1) Massage toward the heart when working below the shoulders. Begin with the part of a limb closest to the heart (i.e., stroke the elbow to the shoulder first; the wrist to the elbow second; the hand third).

2) Massage your neck and head with circular motions, trying to move the skin and soft tissue, not gliding your fingers on the skin.

3) Begin your strokes gently, increasing pressure with each succeeding stroke. Then, lighten your pressure, ending with a smooth, soothing stroke. Relative to the pressure of any given stroke, your touch should always be firmer moving toward the heart, lighter away from the heart.

4) A slower tempo will relax you, a faster tempo will invigorate you. Choose a rhythm appropriate for your particular needs.

Suggested Routine

1) Left arm (elbow to shoulder; elbow in a circular motion; wrist to elbow; knead hand; finish with a stroke of the whole arm upward, then lightly downward).

2) Right arm (following the same directions as the left).

3) Gently massage your abdomen, waist, and sides in an upward circular motion (your right hand going counterclockwise as you look down; your left hand clockwise as you look down).

4) Left leg (knee to buttocks; knee in a circular motion; ankle to knee; knead feet; finish with a stroke of the whole leg upward, then lightly downward).

5) Face (gentle, circular, upward motions).

6) Neck and shoulders (circular, kneading motions).

7) Head (circular motions moving the scalp over the skull).

A.R.E. Press

A.R.E. Press is a publisher and distributor of books, audiotapes, and videos that offer guidance for a more fulfilling life. Our products are based on, or are compatible with, the concepts in the psychic readings of Edgar Cayce.

We especially seek to create products which carry forward the inspirational story of individuals who have made practical application of the Cayce legacy.

For a free catalog, please write to A.R.E. Press at the address below or call toll free 1-800-723-1112. For any other information, please call 804-428-3588, extension 220.

A.R.E. Press
Sixty-Eighth & Atlantic Avenue
P.O. Box 656
Virginia Beach, VA 23451-0656